Published By Adam Gilbin

@ Calvin Shelton

Yoga: Balance for Body, Mind, and Soul

All Right RESERVED

ISBN 978-87-94477-56-7

TABLE OF CONTENTS

chapter 1 1

Type And Best Poses Of Yoga 1

Chapter 2 16

Understanding Yoga Styles And Their Differences 16

Chapter 3 25

Yoga And Meditation: Benefits And Differences 25

Chapter 4 34

Mindful Movement In Daily Life 34

Chapter 5 42

Introduction To Yoga For Stress Relief And Flexibility ... 42

Chapter 6 83

Poses For A Healthy Outer Body 83

Chapter 7 101

Poses For A Healthy Inner Body 101

Chapter 8 114

Characteristics Of Yoga 114

Chapter 9 122

Losing Weight Through Yoga.. 122

Chapter 10 146

Understanding Stress And Its Impact On Your Body.... 146

Chapter 1

Type And Best Poses Of Yoga

Types of yoga

In recent years, yoga has come a long way. Review the timetable for any studio, and you can see all forms of yoga, from aerial Yoga and Acro Yoga to ashtanga yoga and kundalini yoga. Many of the most current and unique variations of the ancient art could have been encountered – or tried – by you, for example, hip hop yoga, HIIT Yoga, and naked yoga.

The many types of yoga are discussed below:

1. Yoga of Vinyasa

Vinyasa is "specifically placed" and Yoga postures in this situation. Vinyasa yoga is the most critical type of yoga, which is usually considered.

How to do it:

In Vinyasa lessons, the breath and movement must be synchronized to float from position to position. The types of Vinyasa can differ depending on the teacher, and in different sequences, there may be multiple poses.

2. Yoga of Hatha

The Sanskrit word "Hatha" is an umbrella term for all physical postures in yoga. In the west, hatha yoga refers to any other kind of yoga that is based on physical activity (Ashtanga, Iyengar). Nevertheless, the different forms of yoga are distinct from traditional yoga exercises, including kriya, raja, and karma yoga. Physical yoga is well known and has many types.

How to perform it:

To beginners, Hatha yoga courses are ideal because they are typically more advanced than other forms of yoga. Today's Hatha classes are a conventional technique for respiration and meditation. When you are new to yoga, hatha yoga is a great start.

3. Yoga Iyengar

The Iyengar Yoga is based on harmonization and thorough and precise movements. In an Iyengar class, students perform some positions during breathing control.

How to do this:

Poses usually last a long time as the poses are changed. Iyengar relies heavily on guidance, which helps students improve their shape and take a healthy approach. While you won't run around, after an Iyengar class, you'll get a training course and feel unbelievably accessible and comfortable. This style is perfect for people with slow and methodical injuries.

4. Yoga of Kundalini

Kundalini yoga is spiritual and physical in equal parts. This style relieves the energy of kundalini in the body that is trapped or enveloped in the lower back.

5. Yoga for Ashtanga

Ashtanga Yoga requires an incredibly physically challenging series of postures, and this yoga style certainly doesn't appeal to beginners. I just enjoy an accomplished yogi. Ashtanga begins with five A sun greetings and five B sun greetings, then transitions into a sequence of floor and standing positions.

6. Yoga for Bikram

Bikram Yoga is named after Bikram Choudhury. Usually, 1050 degrees, 40 percent humidity, of set poses in a sauna-like environment. Choudhury was exposed to sexual abuse and violence in the United States in 2017 and fled to Mexico. To disassociate the creator of several studios, which used to be Bikram, now perform hot yoga.

How we can do it:

A set of 26 essential postures, each performed twice, are part of the series. Many of these positions concentrate on aligning correctly. If you are interested in heat-enhancing yoga, look for a hot-yoga classroom.

7. Yin Yoga Yin

Yin Yoga is a slow pace yoga style that retains sitting positions for more extended periods. Yin may also help you achieve inner peace as a meditative yoga exercise.

How we can do it:

Yin is an excellent class for starting classes since postures can take 45 seconds to 2 minutes. The types are easy since much of the research is meant to be done by you. Find out what you need to know about yin yoga found here, our crash course.

8. Restorative yoga

Restorative yoga focuses on calming down and relaxing the mind after a long day. At the heart of this style is the relaxation of the body. Restorative yoga also helps to purify the mind and release the tension.

How we can do it:

During the yoga exercise, you spend more time at fewer postures. Many of the tasks are changed to make you safer and more straightforward. Like Iyengar, other accessories, such as blankets, bolsters, and pillows, are used and put correctly.

9. Yoga in the Prenatal

Prenatal yoga is mainly for women who are going to be "moms." Some have said that prenatal activities are one of the best kinds of exercise for expectant moms because of work on the pelvic floor. It concentrates on relaxation and bonding with the young infant.

10. Anusara concentrates

Anusara concentrates on spirals and how every part of the body can move and is also recognized because of its emphasis on opening the heart.

BEST POSES OF YOGA

If you are new to yoga, you need to learn those positions so that you can feel relaxed in a class or exercise at home.

It's not easy to restrict anything because, in the physical yoga exercise (asana), there are more than 300 positions, but the following discussion will guide you in the right direction. Whenever you take 5-10 breaths, you can also create a perfect yoga program for beginners for yourself every day.

The best yoga poses are:

Mountain pose

This pose is the basis for all standing poses. It helps you to feel the Earth beneath you to ground in your feet. The location of the mountain can seem like "just standing."

How to do it:

Start to stand together with your feet. At the time of opening them, press all ten toes flat. Keep the quadriceps and bring them up in the inner thighs. Draw in and out your abdominal when lifting your shoulders and force the tops down.

Feel the blades of the arm come over, and the chest open but bring the hands inwards to the body. Just think of a string that pulls the head's crown up to the top and breathe deeply into the abdomen.

Hold 5-8 breaths.

Downward Facing Dog:

For most yogi and yoga exercises, Dog Downward stretches and strengthens the entire body.

How to do this:

Come under your shoulders and knees under your thighs on all fours with your braces. Hang your feet underneath and lift your hips out of the floor as you move them to your knees.

If you have tight hamstrings, keep your knees slightly bent; if you do not want to straighten your legs, keep the hips back. Move your hands forward if you need to invest more time.

Place the palms tightly and tilt the inner elbows to each other. Cut the abdominal holes and tie the legs together to bring the abdomen close to the thighs until you collapse down on your hands and knees for 5-8 breaths to recover.

Plank

Plank shows us how to align our hands with the whole body. It's a perfect way to strengthen the belly and learn to use our breath to help us remain in a tough position.

How to do it?

Slide the heels back enough till you feel like your head is a straight line of energy.

Push the lower abdominals, lift the shoulders off the neck, draw the ribs, breathe in a deep 8-10 respirations.

Triangle:

Triangle is an excellent pose for stretching the sides of the spine, expanding the lungs, strengthening the legs and toning the whole body.

How to do it

Start with one leg apart from your feet. Spread your arms and extend them to the heights of your back. Turn the right foot 90 degrees and the left foot 45 degrees.

Engage your abdominal and quadriceps as you stick across your right hip. Please raise your left arm to a ceiling and put your right hand on your foot, shine, or knee (or a block, if you do have one). Turn your eyes up and keep your eyes 5-8 breaths. Step up on the other side and repeat.

Tree

For newcomers to work on concentration and consistency and how to relax while standing and keeping their corps on one foot balanced. Tree Pose1 helps in outstanding balance.

Go and put the right foot in your upper left inner thigh.

How to do this?

Bring your hands down in prayer and find the place you can hold in a steady gaze before you. Holding 8-10 breaths and then switch sides. Be sure you don't lean to the front and relax your abdominals and shoulders.

Warrior 1

Warrior 1 poses are essential to build strength and endurance in yoga. They give us confidence and expand the hips and thighs while generating power in the bottom body and core.

Warrior 1 is a mild backband; it is an excellent position to stretch open the forebody (quads, hip flexors, psoas). The thighs, arms, ribs, heart, and upper body are strengthened.

What to do: For Warrior One, with your left foot coming to the plunge, you should make a giant move back, followed by a left heel, and turn your left toes forward 75 degrees.

Hold your chest, and underneath press your hands. Put the right leg forward once back.

Warrior 2

Warrior 2 is a hip opener outside, and the inner thighs are extended, and groin extended. With other lateral postures like a triangle, extended angle, and half lunar balance, it is a good starting point.

How to do this: Push one leg apart with your feet. Turn right 90 °, and turn left 45 °, and turn right. Bend the right knee to the right ankle while holding the body between the knees.

Extend your neck and look over your right hand to your hands. Keep 8-10. Keeping your feet on the opposite side before extending the right leg and repeated to the left side.

Seated Forward Bend

Seated Forward Fold It is essential to incorporate a forward bend into the yoga exercise to stretch the hamstrings, the lower sides, and the upper area of the back. It is the perfect fold for everyone to begin to open up their body.

If you feel any sharp pain, you need to go back; but if you feel stress when you fold forward and you can keep breathing, you will slowly begin to loosen up and let go. Furthermore, you can also keep your knees bent in the pose as long as your legs are flexed and together.

How to do it:

start sitting with your legs together, your legs firmly bent and not turning in or out, and your hands beside your hips. Lift your chest and start twisting forward from your waist. You should also Involve your lower abdominals and imagine your belly button moving to the top of your thighs.

Once you've hit your maximum, stop breathing for 8-10 breaths. Make sure your shoulders, your head, and your neck are all free.

Pose of Bridge

Bridget counterposes for a forward bend is a backbend. A bridge is a good beginner's backbend that stretches the front body and strengthens the back.

Ways to do it: you have to lie down on your back and set aside your legs of hip-width. Press your feet firmly and lift your ass off the mat. Put your hands together and press your fists down to the floor as you open your chest even more.

Imagine dragging your heels to your shoulders on the mat to involve your hamstrings. Hold for 8-10 breaths, then lower your hips and repeat for two more times.

Child's Pose

Everyone needs a good rest, and the child's pose is perfect not only for beginners but also for yoga practitioners of all ages.

It is nice to learn how to use the kid pose if you're sick of down dog pose, before you go to bed at night, or if you have a mental break and stress/stress release at any time.

How to do it: Start on all the fours and then join the knees and feet as you sit down the ass and spread the arms out. Slide the head down to the ground (or the pillow or blanket) and release the entire body as long as you want to keep it!

Chapter 2

Understanding Yoga Styles and Their Differences

One of the first steps in your yoga journey is understanding the multitude of yoga styles available. Each style carries its own philosophy, approach, and benefits.

Here, we explore some of the most prominent yoga styles in greater detail:

Iyengar Yoga: This style focuses on precision and alignment, making use of props like belts, blocks, and wall ropes to perform poses with perfect alignment. It's an excellent choice for those who are detail-oriented and looking to refine their postures.

Kundalini Yoga: Known as the "yoga of awareness," Kundalini combines dynamic breathing techniques, meditation, and the chanting of mantras to awaken the Kundalini energy within. It's a holistic approach that delves into the spiritual aspects of yoga.

Yin Yoga: Yin yoga is a slow-paced style where poses are held for extended periods, often up to several minutes. It targets the deep connective tissues, promoting deep stretching and relaxation.

Restorative Yoga: This gentle style uses props to support the body, allowing for deep relaxation. It's ideal for those seeking to de-stress, recover from injuries, or achieve a state of profound relaxation.

Hatha Yoga: Often considered the umbrella term for all physical yoga practices, Hatha yoga is a gentle introduction to the most basic yoga postures. It typically involves a slower-paced, foundational practice that focuses on the alignment of the body, breath, and mind.

Vinyasa Yoga: Known for its dynamic and flowing sequences, Vinyasa yoga links breath with movement. It's a physically demanding style that emphasizes the importance of synchronized breathing and continuous motion.

Ashtanga Yoga: Ashtanga is a vigorous style of yoga that follows a specific sequence of postures and is similar to Vinyasa but faster-paced and more intense. It's often preferred by those seeking a more challenging and structured practice.

Bikram Yoga: Conducted in a room heated to a high temperature, Bikram yoga involves a series of 26 challenging poses and two breathing exercises. The heat is believed to enhance flexibility and detoxification.

By exploring these diverse yoga styles, you gain insight into the rich tapestry of practices and philosophies available. It's essential to align your chosen style with your goals, physical condition, and preferences.

Yoga Equipment and Clothing: Enhancing Your Practice

While yoga is a minimalistic practice in terms of required equipment, having the right gear can significantly enhance your experience. Here's a closer look at the essential yoga equipment and clothing:

Yoga Attire: Comfortable, breathable clothing is the key to a productive practice. It should allow free movement and flexibility. Additionally, consider clothing that suits the room's temperature, as yoga studios may vary in temperature and humidity.

Meditation Cushion: If your practice includes meditation, a cushion or zafu can provide a comfortable and supportive seat, allowing you to maintain a seated position for longer periods without discomfort.

Water Bottle: Staying hydrated during your practice is crucial. Having a water bottle nearby ensures you can replenish fluids as needed, especially during more vigorous sessions.

Towel: In heated yoga styles like Bikram, a towel can be invaluable for absorbing sweat and providing a non-slip surface, enhancing your safety and comfort during practice.

Yoga Mat: A quality yoga mat provides a stable, comfortable surface for your practice. It offers grip and cushioning to support your poses while also creating a dedicated space for your practice.

Yoga Props: Depending on your chosen style, you may need props like blocks, straps, bolsters, and blankets. These props assist with alignment and comfort during poses, ensuring that you can achieve postures with precision.

By investing in the appropriate gear, you not only ensure your comfort and safety but also create a dedicated space for your practice, both mentally and physically.

Yoga Etiquette: Fostering Harmony and Respect

Yoga is not only a personal journey but also a shared experience when practiced in a group setting. Observing yoga etiquette is crucial in creating a harmonious and respectful environment for all practitioners. Here are some common elements of yoga etiquette:

Punctuality: Arriving on time is essential. Being punctual ensures you have sufficient time to settle in and prevents disruption once the class begins. Tardiness can disrupt the **Personal Hygiene**: Practicing good personal hygiene is a sign of respect for yourself and others. Clean clothing and the use of natural deodorant can help maintain a pleasant practice environment.

Respect for Space: Mindful positioning of your mat and your proximity to others is crucial.

Ensure that there's sufficient room for everyone and that you respect the space of your fellow practitioners.

Savasana: Staying for Savasana, the final relaxation pose, is essential. This closing pose allows you to integrate the benefits of your practice and shows respect for the teacher and fellow students. Leaving early disrupts the tranquility of the practice space.

Clean Up: After your practice, neatly stow your equipment, cleaning and sanitizing it as needed. This simple act of tidying up respects the studio's cleanliness and order.

of the class and the focus of other practitioners.

Shoes Off: Most yoga studios require removing your shoes before entering the practice area. This simple gesture shows respect for the sacred space of the studio.

Silence Your Phone: To avoid interruptions, turn off your mobile phone or switch it to silent mode before entering the studio. The distractions of ringing phones can disrupt the peaceful atmosphere.

By adhering to these basic principles of yoga etiquette, you not only respect the environment but also enhance your overall yoga experience. The yoga studio becomes a sanctuary where practitioners come together in a shared journey of self-discovery, and each individual's adherence to etiquette contributes to a harmonious and respectful atmosphere.

In summary, understanding and embracing "Yoga Basics" are the cornerstones of a fulfilling yoga practice. As you delve into the world of yoga styles, equip yourself with the right gear, and observe yoga etiquette, you lay a solid foundation for your yoga journey. Whether you're a beginner or an experienced yogi, the basics remain a touchstone, ensuring that your practice remains rooted in tradition and guided by respect and mindfulness

Chapter 3

YOGA AND MEDITATION: BENEFITS AND DIFFERENCES

The first known record of meditation and yoga meditation as disciplines dates back more than 5000 years. Both yoga and meditation practices originated in northern India; we know this because both yoga and meditation are mentioned in some very old texts which are known as the Rig Veda.

It is estimated that today, the physical practice of yoga and meditation are regularly engaged in by more than 500 million people worldwide. That's a lot of people with benefits of group meditation. Maybe they knew something we don't. Let's find out, shall we?

The physical aspect of yoga and meditation can be combined with controlled breathing. Doing this while keeping your eyes closed to focus attention, can be a very powerful tool. Additionally, the therapeutic benefits of yoga and yoga meditation can assist in the reduction in the severity of some physical issues such as hypertension, sleep problems and anxiety, all the while building a stronger immune system. It's all good.

Mindfulness Meditation Meaning

The term "mindfulness" is used here in conjunction with meditation, and simply means the focus of attention on an activity you are doing in the present moment. Mindful meditation yoga is achieving a meditative state through the practice of mindfulness meditation can also help calm some common chronic mental health issues that occur, especially to those new to addiction recovery, such as anxiety and depression. It is for this reason that mindfulness meditation is highly recommended.

Reduction of stress is extremely vital to our overall health. Because we live in a very high demand, high stress world, developing the ability to occasionally relax our body and mind once in a while are more important than ever.

The term chronic, as used here, means the condition has lasted for a while or seems to recur regularly. Chronic stress is considered to be a serious health issue, and is known to cause other more serious conditions such as high blood pressure, heart disease, obesity, diabetes, and arthritis.

Yoga Vs Meditation

Some additional benefits of a regular meditation practice include, but are not limited to, a sense of well being. This in turn can generate a feeling of self-acceptance or a capacity for self-love. This too is a vital ingredient for someone new in recovery.

It has been said that one of the first benefits of meditation is emotional sobriety, a quality sorely lacking in many individuals, especially those new to addiction recovery. If you don't believe that, see how far you get driving the speed limit on the freeway of your choice, before being approached by someone who, more likely than not, is lacking in this quality.

Meditate for Spirituality

Yoga versus meditation can be the key that unlocks the mysterious dimension of spirit we all posses. Luckily for many of us in recovery there is no mandate about the type of spirituality we find.

Meditation is a way to calm our overworked nervous system and lessen the constant river of mental activity we all suffer from. In this way, we are more able to explore our inner selves. Some refer to this practice as yoga mindful meditation.

Daily life

Addiction recovery is the process by which we discover who we really are underneath the façade we present to the world to try and fool ourselves or others that we are OK.

There can be too much static and noise in our daily lives. Meditation can be the way to discover and accept ourselves. Through the practice of meditation, we get in touch with our inner selves, or spirit, if you will. This work is actually what is commonly referred to as the "spiritual aspect" of recovery.

Reducing stress

Beginning a mindfulness meditation practice in order to slow our thought process will almost immediately produce a reduction in our stress level, which also has a positive effect on our overactive nervous system.

Improving our ability to focus on the present moment also allows us to experience the pleasant physical sensations of peace we begin to experience through mindfulness meditation.

Focus the "monkey mind"

As stated previously, calming the body and mind through meditation helps to increase our ability to focus and concentrate. Our minds can sometimes behave like agitated monkeys, swinging quickly from worry to guilt to shame, and then back again.

This lack of concentration can limit our ability to focus these overactive "monkey minds" we have. This can, in turn, drastically decrease energy levels, and our experience of the present moment. Seeing as how the present moment is where everything happens, you may not want to miss it.

Yoga and Breath Work

Pranayama practice is one method that can be employed to calm the mind. The word Pranayama is from Sanskrit and literally means regulation of the breath. Control of the breath is one of the main components of both yoga and meditation.

Try using pranayama if you find yourself ruminating, or are having trouble moving on from a negative space. When you find yourself lost in thought, you can come back to the present moment any time. Try using controlled breath to achieve a relaxed state, especially when you may be feeling 'Hangry,' (hungry/angry).

The idea here is to breathe in for a count of five, let's say. Then hold it for a count of five, then release for the same length. Repeat this several times. Try it, it really works!

Seated meditation practice

The act of meditating is usually depicted wherein the individual sits cross legged on the floor, or a cushion. However, those of us with bad joints have found it is also possible to meditate successfully while comfortably seated in a chair. Or even lying down. So, no worries there.

Asana practice

The word Asana simply refers to a specific body posture, and was originally used to indicate a sitting meditation pose. Now, the term Asana can mean any physical pose such as sun salutations (Google it) or any other body position held either during meditation or while engaged in yoga.

Asana Practice during meditation can involve either sitting, standing, lying down or walking. But that's it. So driving, eating, surfing the internet or watching TV do not count.

Chapter 4

Mindful Movement in Daily Life

Mindful Movement in Daily Life: Cultivating Inner Connection through Simple Yoga Practices

In our fast-paced and hectic lives, staying connected with ourselves and maintaining a sense of inner peace can be challenging. Mindful movement, rooted in yoga principles, offers a transformative approach to integrate yoga into our daily routines. By incorporating simple, conscious movements like mindful stretching and walking, we can cultivate a deeper connection with ourselves throughout the day. These practices allow us to foster mindfulness, reduce stress, and enhance our overall well-being, even amidst the busiest of schedules.

The Essence of Mindful Movement

Mindful movement is the art of moving with awareness and intention. It involves practising yoga-inspired movements in a mindful and focused manner. This type of movement encourages individuals to be fully present in the moment, paying attention to their body, breath, and sensations. By bringing mindfulness to daily activities, we can transform ordinary routines into opportunities for self-discovery and inner connection.

Mindful Stretching

Mindful stretching involves a series of gentle yoga-inspired stretches performed with full awareness. The practice focuses on slowly and deliberately moving through various poses, paying attention to the body's sensations and limitations. Mindful stretching not only improves flexibility and relieves tension but also brings a sense of calmness and presence to the mind.

Benefits of Mindful Stretching:

improved Flexibility :

Regular mindful stretching increases flexibility and range of motion in the muscles and joints.

Stress Reduction :

The slow and deliberate nature of mindful stretching promotes relaxation and reduces stress levels.

Enhanced Body Awareness : **Practising mindful stretching cultivates a deeper understanding of the body's needs and limitations.**

Mind-Body Connection :

By being fully present during the practice, individuals strengthen the connection between their body and mind.

Conscious Walking

Conscious walking is a simple yet powerful practice that involves walking with awareness and intention. While walking, practitioners focus on each step, the sensation of the ground beneath their feet, and the rhythm of their breath. Conscious walking can be done anywhere, making it a convenient way to incorporate mindfulness into daily life.

Benefits of Conscious Walking:

Mindfulness on the Go : Co

nscious walking allows individuals to practise mindfulness while going about their daily activities.

Stress Relief:

Focusing on each step and breath helps reduce stress and promotes a sense of calmness.

Connection with Nature :

Conscious walking outdoors enables a deeper connection with nature and the surrounding environment.

Grounding and Centering :

The practice of conscious walking helps ground and centre the mind, promoting mental clarity.

Mindful Breathing

Mindful breathing is a foundational aspect of mindful movement. It involves bringing attention to the breath and observing its natural rhythm without attempting to control it. The breath becomes an anchor, bringing the mind back to the present moment whenever it wanders.

Benefits of Mindful Breathing:

Stress Reduction :

Mindful breathing activates the relaxation response, reducing stress and anxiety levels.

Improved Focus:

The practice enhances concentration and mental clarity.

Emotional Regulation :

Mindful breathing helps individuals manage emotions and reactions more effectively.

Mindfulness in Daily Activities:

By incorporating mindful breathing into daily tasks, individuals stay present and attentive.

Mindful Posture and Alignment

Mindful posture and alignment involve maintaining awareness of body posture throughout the day. Whether sitting at a desk or standing in line, practitioners make a conscious effort to align their body correctly to avoid strain and tension.

Benefits of Mindful Posture and Alignment:

Pain Prevention :

Mindful posture helps prevent back, neck, and shoulder pain caused by poor alignment.

Increased Energy and Vitality :

Proper alignment allows for efficient energy flow throughout the body.

Mindful Presence :

Being mindful of posture brings attention to the present moment and helps break the cycle of unconscious habits.

Incorporating Mindful Movement into Daily Life

Start Small :

Begin with short mindful movement sessions and gradually increase the duration as the practice becomes more comfortable.

Set Reminders :

Use reminders or cues throughout the day to bring attention back to mindful movement and breathing.

Be Kind to Yourself :

Embrace imperfections and avoid self-judgement during the practice. Mindful movement is about cultivating awareness, not achieving perfection.

Create Rituals :

Designate specific times of the day for mindful movement, such as stretching before bed or conscious walking during lunch breaks.

Chapter 5

Introduction to Yoga for Stress Relief and Flexibility

The Power of Yoga in Your Hands

Yoga, often thought of as an exercise routine, is much more than just a physical practice. It's a lifestyle, a philosophy, and a path to serenity that has the potential to change your life. In this chapter, we'll embark on a journey to understand what yoga is, why it's so powerful, and how it can help you combat stress and enhance flexibility.

The Essence of Yoga

Yoga, derived from the Sanskrit word "yuj," which means to unite or yoke, is an ancient practice that dates back thousands of years. It's more than just a form of exercise; it's a holistic approach to well-being that encompasses physical postures, breathing techniques, meditation, and philosophy. The essence of yoga lies in the union of mind, body, and spirit.

A Comprehensive Practice

One of the remarkable aspects of yoga is its comprehensive nature. It's not limited to physical movements or flexibility; it's about integrating various facets of your being. Let's take a closer look at the components that make up this profound practice:

Asanas (Physical Postures): Yoga postures, or asanas, are the most visible aspect of yoga. These postures aim to increase you
r physical flexibility, strength, and balance. They also promote relaxation and reduce tension in your body.

Pranayama (Breathing Techniques):
The breath is considered the bridge between the body and the mind in yoga. Pranayama focuses

on controlling the breath to calm the mind, improve concentration, and reduce stress.

Dhyana (Meditation):
Meditation in yoga is about achieving a state of mental clarity, focus, and inner peace. It's a practice that allows you to quiet the mind and experience a profound sense of tranquility.

Yama and Niyama (Ethical Principles):
Yoga is not just about what you do on the mat; it's about how you live your life. The ethical principles of yoga, known as yama and niyama, guide practitioners to live with integrity, kindness, and self-discipline.

Philosophy:
Yoga has a rich philosophical tradition that delves into the nature of reality, human suffering, and the path to liberation. Understanding this

philosophy can deepen your practice and provide insights into the mind-body connection.

Stress Relief and Flexibility

So, how does yoga address stress relief and flexibility? The physical postures, or asanas, work on stretching and strengthening your muscles, which can help you release physical tension and enhance flexibility. Moreover, they improve blood circulation, which can reduce stress and increase your energy levels.

Beyond the physical, yoga's emphasis on mindfulness, deep breathing, and meditation techniques equips you with invaluable tools to tackle stress at its root. The practice encourages you to be present in the moment, letting go of worries about the past or future. This mental clarity and emotional balance help you navigate life's challenges with ease.

Your Journey Begins

Your journey to stress relief and flexibility starts here. In the chapters to come, we will delve deeper into each aspect of yoga, providing you with practical guidance, expert insights, and step-by-step instructions to incorporate yoga into your life. Whether you're a complete beginner or someone with prior experience, "Yoga for Serenity" will serve as your comprehensive guide. But remember, yoga is not a destination; it's a journey. It's about progress, not perfection. As you embrace this practice, you'll find that the benefits extend far beyond the mat. They ripple into your daily life, transforming the way you handle stress, approach challenges, and experience flexibility in both your body and mind. The path to serenity awaits. Are you ready to step onto the mat and begin your transformative journey? In the following chapters, we'll equip you with the knowledge and techniques you need to unlock the power of yoga and embrace a life of serenity, stress relief, and flexibility.

BEGINNING YOUR WORKOUT

We use the word "workout" loosely here because, as we've pointed out, yoga is less workout and more mind-body exploration. Workout implies sweating as you push your body into exercise mode. That isn't what yoga is about.

So, here's a good way to start your yoga plan. Do these exercises in the order given for a good beginning workout.

Easy Pose

Begin with the easy pose. Easy pose is a comfortable seated position for meditation. This pose opens the hips, lengthens the spine and promotes grounding and inner calm. Basically, you're sitting cross legged like you did in school as a young child. "Criss cross apple sauce", as my teacher used to say!

With the buttocks on the floor, cross your legs and place your feet directly below your knees. Rest your hands on your knees with the palms facing up. Press your hip bones down into the floor and reach the crown of the head up to lengthen the spine. Drop your shoulders down and back and press your chest towards the front of the room.

Relax your face, jaw, and belly. Let your tongue rest on the roof of your mouth just behind your front teeth. Breathe deeply through the nose down into the belly and hold as long as is comfortable.

Downward-Facing Dog

After the easy pose, move into downward-facing dog. This is one of the most widely recognized yoga poses. Downward-Facing Dog is an all-over, rejuvenating stretch.

Benefits include:

Calms the brain and helps relieve stress and mild depression

Relieves menstrual discomfort when done with head supported

Helps prevent osteoporosis Improves digestion

Relieves headache, insomnia, back pain, and fatigue

Therapeutic for high blood pressure, asthma, flat feet, sciatica, sinusitis

Stretches the shoulders, hamstrings, calves, arches, and hands

Strengthens the arms and legs

Helps relieve the symptoms of menopause

Use caution doing this pose if you have carpal tunnel syndrome, are in the late stages of pregnancy, or suffer from high blood pressure.

Come onto the floor on your hands and knees. Set your knees directly below your hips and your hands slightly forward of your shoulders. Spread your palms, index fingers parallel or slightly turned out, and turn your toes under.

Exhale and lift your knees away from the floor. At first keep the knees slightly bent and the heels lifted away from the floor. Lengthen your tailbone away from the back of your pelvis and press it lightly toward the pubis. Against this resistance, lift the sitting bones toward the ceiling, and from your inner ankles draw the inner legs up into the groins.

Then with an exhalation, push your top thighs back and stretch your heels onto or down toward the floor. Straighten your knees but be sure not to lock them. Firm the outer thighs and roll the upper thighs inward slightly. Narrow the front of the pelvis.

Firm the outer arms and press the bases of the index fingers actively into the floor. From these two points, lift along your inner arms from the wrists to the tops of the shoulders. Firm your shoulder blades against your back then widen them and draw them toward the tailbone. Keep the head between the upper arms; don't let it hang.

Stay in this pose anywhere from 1 to 3 minutes. Then bend your knees to the floor with an exhalation and rest.

Sun Salutations

On days when you think you have no time for yoga, try and do at least one or two rounds of the Sun Salutation. You'll feel the difference.

After downward-facing dog, move into 3 rounds of sun salutations.

Stand facing the direction of the sun with both feet touching. Bring the hands together, palm-to-palm, at the heart. Inhale and raise the arms upward. Slowly bend backward, stretching arms above the head. Exhale slowly bending forward, touching the earth with respect until the hands are in line with the feet, head touching knees.

Inhale and move the right leg back away from the body in a wide backward step. Keep the hands and feet firmly on the ground, with the left foot between the hands. Raise the head. While exhaling, bring the left foot together with the right.

Keep arms straight, raise the hips and align the head with the arms, forming an upward arch.

Exhale and lower the body to the floor until the feet, knees, hands, chest, and forehead are touching the ground. Inhale and slowly raise the head and bend backward as much as possible, bending the spine to the maximum

While exhaling, bring the left foot together with the right. Keep arms straight, raise the hips and align the head with the arms, forming an upward arch. Inhale and move the right leg back away from the body in a wide backward step.

Keep the hands and feet firmly on the ground, with the left foot between the hands. Raise the head. Exhale slowly bending forward, touching the earth with respect until the hands are in line with the feet, head touching knees.

Inhale and raise the arms upward. Slowly bend backward, stretching arms above the head. Stand facing the direction of the sun with both feet touching. Bring the hands together, palm-to-palm, at the heart.

The sequence will look something like this:

Tree Pose - Vriksha Asana

Benefits include:

Strengthens thighs, calves, ankles, and spine
Stretches the groins and inner thighs, chest and shoulders
Improves sense of balance
Relieves sciatica and reduces flat feet

Use caution if you suffer from insomnia or low blood pressure. If you have high blood pressure, do not raise your arms above your head.
Stand with the feet together and the arms by your sides. Bend the right leg at the knee, raise the right thigh and bring the sole of the right foot as high up the inside of the left thigh as possible.

Balancing on the left foot, raise both arms over the head, keep the elbows unbent and join the palms together. Hold the posture while breathing gently through the nostrils for about 10 complete breaths.

Lower the arms and right leg and return to the tad-asana, standing position with feet together and arms at the sides. Pause for a few moments and repeat on the opposite leg. Do this two or three times per leg or as long as is comfortable.

The challenge of the vriksha-asana is maintaining balance on one leg. Poor balance is often the result of a restless mind or distracted attention. Regular practice of this posture will help focus the mind and cultivate concentration (dharana). When practicing vriksha-asana it may help to imagine or picture a tree in the mind and apply the following technique: Imagine that the foot you are balanced on is the root of the tree and the leg is the trunk.

Continue by imagining the head and outstretched arms as the branches and leaves of the tree. You may be unsteady for a while and find the body swaying back and forth, but don't break the concentration. Like a tree bending in the wind and yet remaining upright, the body can maintain balance.

Aim to achieve the "rootedness" and firmness of a tree. Regular practice of the vriksha-asana improves concentration, balance and coordination. Because the weight of the entire body is balanced on one foot, the muscles of that leg are strengthened and toned as well.

As you advance in this posture and are able to remain standing for more than a few moments, try closing the eyes and maintaining your balance.

Extended Triangle Pose

Benefits include:

- Stretches and strengthens the thighs, knees, and ankles
- Stretches the hips, groins, hamstrings, and calves; shoulders, chest, and spine
- Stimulates the abdominal organs
- Helps relieve stress
- Improves digestion
- Helps relieve the symptoms of menopause
- Relieves backache, especially through second trimester of pregnancy
- Therapeutic for anxiety, flat feet, infertility, neck pain, osteoporosis, and sciatica

Use caution if you suffer from low blood pressure, have a heart condition, or have neck problems.

Stand with the feet together and the arms by your sides. Separate the feet slightly further than shoulder distance apart. Inhale and raise both arms straight out from the shoulders parallel to the floor with the palms facing down.

Exhale slowly while turning the torso to the left, bend at the waist and bring the right hand down to the left ankle. The palm of the right hand is placed along the outside of the left ankle. The left arm should be extended upward. Both legs and arms are kept straight without bending the knees and elbows.

Turn the head upward to the left and gaze up at the fingertips of the left hand. Inhale and return to a standing position with the arms outstretched. Hold this position for the duration of the exhaled breath. Exhale and repeat on the opposite side.

The triangle pose is basically doing slow toe touches while concentrating on your breathing and stretching your body.

Seated Forward Bend – Paschimottanasana

Literally translated as "intense stretch of the west," Paschimottanasana can help a distracted mind unwind.

Benefits include:

• Calms the brain and helps relieve stress and mild depression

• Stretches the spine, shoulders, hamstrings

• Stimulates the liver, kidneys, ovaries, and uterus

• Improves digestion

• Helps relieve the symptoms of menopause and menstrual discomfort

• Soothes headache and anxiety and reduces fatigue

- Therapeutic for high blood pressure, infertility, insomnia, and sinusitis
- Traditional texts say that Paschimottanasana increases appetite, reduces obesity, and cures diseases.

Use caution if you suffer from asthma or have a back injury.

Sit on the floor with your buttocks supported on a folded blanket and your legs straight in front of you. Press actively through your heels. Rock slightly onto your left buttock, and pull your right sitting bone away from the heel with your right hand. Repeat on the other side.

Turn the top thighs in slightly and press them down into the floor. Press through your palms or finger tips on the floor beside your hips and lift the top of the sternum toward the ceiling as the top thighs descend.

Draw the inner groins deep into the pelvis. Inhale, and keeping the front torso long, lean forward from the hip joints, not the waist. Lengthen the tailbone away from the back of your pelvis. If possible take the sides of the feet with your hands, thumbs on the soles, elbows fully extended; if this isn't possible, loop a strap around the foot soles, and hold the strap firmly. Be sure your elbows are straight, not bent.

When you are ready to go further, don't forcefully pull yourself into the forward bend, whether your hands are on the feet or holding the strap. Always lengthen the front torso into the pose, keeping your head raised.

If you are holding the feet, bend the elbows out to the sides and lift them away from the floor; if holding the strap, lighten your grip and walk the hands forward, keeping the arms long. The lower belly should touch the thighs first, and then the upper belly, then the ribs, and the head last.

With each inhalation, lift and lengthen the front torso just slightly; with each exhalation release a little more fully into the forward bend. In this way the torso oscillates and lengthens almost imperceptibly with the breath. Eventually you may be able to stretch the arms out beyond the feet on the floor.

Stay in the pose anywhere from 1 to 3 minutes. To come up, first lift the torso away from the thighs and straighten the elbows again if they are bent. Then inhale and lift the torso up by pulling the tailbone down and into the pelvis.

Bound Angle *Pose* - Baddha Konasana

Bound Angle Pose, also called Cobbler's Pose after the typical sitting position of Indian cobblers, is an excellent groin and hip-opener. Benefits include:

• Stimulates abdominal organs, ovaries and prostate gland, bladder, and kidneys

- Stimulates the heart and improves general circulation
- Stretches the inner thighs, groins, and knees
- Helps relieve mild depression, anxiety, and fatigue
- Soothes menstrual discomfort and sciatica
- Helps relieve the symptoms of menopause
- Therapeutic for flat feet, high blood pressure, infertility, and asthma
- Consistent practice of this pose until late into pregnancy is said to help ease childbirth.
- Traditional texts say that Baddha Konasana destroys disease and gets rid of fatigue.

Sit with your legs straight out in front of you, raising your pelvis on a blanket if your hips or groins are tight. Exhale, bend your knees, pull your heels toward your pelvis, then drop your knees out to the sides and press the soles of your feet together.

Bring your heels as close to your pelvis as you comfortably can. With the first and second finger and thumb, grasp the big toe of each foot. Always keep the outer edges of the feet firmly on the floor. If it isn't possible to hold the toes, clasp each hand around the same-side ankle or shin. Sit so that the pubis in front and the tailbone in back are equidistant from the floor. The perineum then will be approximately parallel to the floor and the pelvis in a neutral position. Firm the sacrum and shoulder blades against the back and lengthen the front torso through the top of the sternum.

Never force your knees down. Instead release the heads of the thigh bones toward the floor. When this action leads, the knees follow.

Stay in this pose anywhere from 1 to 5 minutes. Then inhale, lift your knees away from the floor, and extend the legs back to their original position.

Wide-Angle Seated Forward Bend - Upavistha Konasana

Upavistha Konasana is a good preparation for most of the seated forward bends and twists, as well as the wide-leg standing poses

Benefits include:

- Stretches the insides and backs of the legs
- Stimulates the abdominal organs
- Strengthens the spine
- Calms the brain
- Releases groins

Use caution with this exercise if you have a lower back injury.

Sit with your legs extended out in front of you, then lean your torso back slightly on your hands and lift and open your legs to an angle of about 90 degrees (the legs should form an approximate right angle, with the pubis at the apex). Press your hands against the floor and slide your buttocks forward, widening the legs another 10 to 20 degrees. If you can't sit comfortably on the floor, raise your buttocks on a folded blanket. Rotate your thighs outwardly, pinning the outer thighs against the floor, so that the knee caps point straight up toward the ceiling. Reach out through your heels and stretch your soles, pressing though the balls of the feet.

With your thigh bones pressed heavily into the floor and your knee caps pointing up at the ceiling, walk your hands forward between your legs. Keep your arms long.

As with all forward bends, the emphasis is on moving from the hip joints and maintaining the length of the front torso. As soon as you find yourself bending from the waist, stop, re-establish the length from the pubis to the navel, and continue forward if possible.

Increase the forward bend on each exhalation until you feel a comfortable stretch in the backs of your legs. Stay in the pose 1 minute or longer. Then come up on an inhalation with a long front torso.

Full Boat Pose

An abdominal and deep hip flexor strengthener, Boat Pose requires you to balance on the tripod of your sitting bones and tailbone.

Benefits include:

• Strengthens the abdomen, hip flexors, and spine

• Stimulates the kidneys, thyroid and prostate glands, and intestines

• Helps relieve stress

• Improves digestion

Use caution if you have low blood pressure, insomnia, neck problems, are pregnant or menstruating.

Sit on the floor with your legs straight in front of you. Press your hands on the floor a little behind your hips, fingers pointing toward the feet, and strengthen the arms. Lift through the top of the sternum and lean back slightly. As you do this make sure your back doesn't round; continue to lengthen the front of your torso between the pubis and top sternum. Sit on the "tripod" of your two sitting bones and tailbone.

Exhale and bend your knees, then lift your feet off the floor, so that the thighs are angled about 45-50 degrees relative to the floor. Lengthen your tailbone into the floor and lift your pubis toward your navel. If possible, slowly straighten your knees, raising the tips of your toes slightly above the level of your eyes. If this isn't possible remain with your knees bent, perhaps lifting the shins parallel to the floor.

Stretch your arms alongside the legs, parallel to each other and the floor. Spread the shoulder blades across your back and reach strongly out through the fingers. If this isn't possible, keep the hands on the floor beside your hips or hold on to the backs of your thighs.

While the lower belly should be firm, it shouldn't get hard and thick. Try to keep the lower belly relatively flat. Press the heads of the thigh bones toward the floor to help anchor the pose and lift the top sternum. Breathe easily. Tip the chin slightly toward the sternum so the base of the skull lifts lightly away from the back of the neck. At first stay in the pose for 10-20 seconds. Gradually increase the time of your stay to 1 minute. Release the legs with an exhalation and sit upright on an inhalation.

Bridge Pose

This active version of Bridge Pose calms the brain and rejuvenates tired legs.

Benefits include:

• Stretches the chest, neck, and spine

• Calms the brain and helps alleviate stress and mild depression

• Stimulates abdominal organs, lungs, and thyroid

• Rejuvenates tired legs

• Improves digestion

• Helps relieve the symptoms of menopause

• Relieves menstrual discomfort when done supported

• Reduces anxiety, fatigue, backache, headache, and insomnia

• Therapeutic for asthma, high blood pressure, osteoporosis, and sinusitis Use caution if you have a neck injury.

Lie supine on the floor, and if necessary, place a thickly folded blanket under your shoulders to protect your neck. Bend your knees and set your feet on the floor, heels as close to the sitting bones as possible.

Exhale and, pressing your inner feet and arms actively into the floor, push your tailbone upward toward the pubis, firming (but not hardening) the buttocks, and lift the buttocks off the floor. Keep your thighs and inner feet parallel. Clasp the hands below your pelvis and extend through the arms to help you stay on the tops of your shoulders.

Lift your buttocks until the thighs are about parallel to the floor. Keep your knees directly over the heels, but push them forward, away from the hips, and lengthen the tailbone toward the backs of the knees. Lift the pubis toward the navel.

Lift your chin slightly away from the sternum and, firming the shoulder blades against your back, press the top of the sternum toward the chin. Firm the outer arms, broaden the shoulder blades, and try to lift the space between them at the base of the neck (where it's resting on the blanket) up into the torso.

Stay in the pose anywhere from 30 seconds to 1 minute. Release with an exhalation, rolling the spine slowly down onto the floor.

Legs-Up-the-Wall Pose - Viparita Karani

Said to reverse the normal downward flow of a precious subtle fluid called amrita (immortal) or soma (extract) in the Hatha Yoga Pradipika, modern yogis agree that Viparita Karani may have the power to cure whatever ails you.

Benefits include:

- Relieves tired or cramped legs and feet

- Gently stretches the back legs, front torso, and the back of the neck
- Relieves mild backache
-

Calms the mind

The pose described this is a passive, supported variation of the shoulder stand. For your support you'll need one or two thickly folded blankets or a firm round bolster. You'll also need to rest your legs vertically (or nearly so) on a wall or other upright support.

Before performing the pose, determine two things about your support: its height and its distance from the wall. If you're stiffer, the support should be lower and placed farther from the wall; if you're more flexible, use a higher support that is closer to the wall.

Your distance from the wall also depends on your height: if you're shorter move closer to the wall, if taller move farther from the wall. Experiment with the position of your support until you find the placement that works for you.

Start with your support about 5 to 6 inches away from the wall. Sit sideways on right end of the support, with your right side against the wall (left-handers can substitute "left" for "right" in these instructions). Exhale and, with one smooth movement, swing your legs up onto the wall and your shoulders and head lightly down onto the floor.

The first few times you do this you may slide off the support and plop down with your buttocks on the floor. Don't get discouraged. Try lowering the support and/or moving it slightly further off the wall until you gain some facility with this movement, then move back closer to the wall.

Your sitting bones don't need to be right against the wall, but they should be "dripping" down into the space between the support and the wall.

Check that the front of your torso gently arches from the pubis to the top of the shoulders.

If the front of your torso seems flat, then you've probably slipped a bit off the support. Bend your knees, press your feet into the wall and lift your pelvis off the support a few inches, tuck the support a little higher up under your pelvis, then lower your pelvis onto the support again.

Lift and release the base of your skull away from the back of your neck and soften your throat. Don't push your chin against your sternum; instead let your sternum lift toward the chin. Take a small roll (made from a towel for example) under your neck if the cervical spine feels flat. Open your shoulder blades away from the spine and release your hands and arms out to your sides, palms up.

Keep your legs relatively firm, just enough to hold them vertically in place. Release the heads of the thigh bones and the weight of your belly deeply into your torso, toward the back of the pelvis. Soften your eyes and turn them down to look into your heart.

Stay in this pose anywhere from 5 to 15 minutes. Be sure not to twist off the support when coming out. Instead, slide off the support onto the floor before turning to the side. You can also bend your knees and push your feet against the wall to lift your pelvis off the support. Then slide the support to one side, lower your pelvis to the floor, and turn to the side. Stay on your side for a few breaths, and come up to sitting with an exhalation.

Corpse Pose - Savasana

Savasana is a pose of total relaxation making it one of the most challenging asanas.

Benefits include:

- Calms the brain and helps relieve stress and mild depression
- Relaxes the body
- Reduces headache, fatigue, and insomnia

- Helps to lower blood pressure

In Savasana it's essential that the body be placed in a neutral position. Sit on the floor with your knees bent, feet on the floor, and lean back onto your forearms. Lift your pelvis slightly off the floor and, with your hands, push the back of the pelvis toward the tailbone, then return the pelvis to the floor.

Inhale and slowly extend the right leg, then the left, pushing through the heels. Release both legs, softening the groins, and see that the legs are angled evenly relative to the mid-line of the torso, and that the feet turn out equally. You should narrow the front pelvis and soften (but don't flatten) the lower back.

With your hands lift the base of the skull away from the back of the neck and release the back of the neck down toward the tailbone. If you have any difficulty doing this, support the back of the head and neck on a folded blanket. Broaden the base of the skull too, and lift the crease of the neck diagonally into the center of the head. Make sure your ears are equidistant from your shoulders.

Reach your arms toward the ceiling, perpendicular to the floor. Rock slightly from side to side and broaden the back ribs and the shoulder blades away from the spine. Then release the arms to the floor, angled evenly relative to the mid-line of torso.

Turn the arms outward and stretch them away from the space between the shoulder blades. Rest the backs of the hands on the floor as close as you comfortably can to the index finger knuckles. Make sure the shoulder blades are resting evenly on the floor. Imagine the lower tips of the shoulder blades are lifting diagonally into your back toward the top of the sternum. From here, spread the collarbones.

In addition to quieting the physical body in Savasana, it's also necessary to pacify the sense organs. Soften the root of the tongue, the wings of the nose, the channels of the inner ears, and the skin of the forehead, especially around the bridge of the nose between the eyebrows. Let the eyes sink to the back of the head, then turn them downward to gaze at the heart. Release your brain to the back of the head.

Stay in this pose for 5 minutes for every 30 minutes of practice. To exit, first roll gently with an exhalation onto one side, preferably the right. Take 2 or 3 breaths. With another exhalation press your hands against the floor and lift your torso, dragging your head slowly after. The head should always come up last.

After completing these exercises, take a few moments to practice some deep meditation which is covered in the next section.

Chapter 6

Poses for A Healthy Outer Body

As time goes on, more and more people are realizing and experiencing the benefits of yoga first hand. There are so many reasons why yoga has been a main form of exercise and movement for hundreds and thousands of years; perhaps one of the most prominent reasons in today's society is weight loss. There is no doubt that, in today's world, obesity is an epidemic. Being overweight may cause a host of other chronic issues and complications that may become life-threatening. In order to lose weight, we must educate ourselves on healthy practices. Yoga is one such practice, because *anybody* can participate in it and reap the benefits therefrom. The following postures will challenge your physical strength. They will help you to lose weight and tone the body, especially if practiced regularly. Take each posture slowly and at your own pace. Before you know it, you'll be a pro!

1. Boat Pose (Paripurna Navasana)

Begin in a seated position with both feet planted on the floor. Place your hands on the mat behind your hips, fingertips pointing towards the feet. Take a few deep breaths to release any tension in the back. When you feel ready, exhale and lift your feet up off the ground, extending the legs fully. If you can, double check to make sure the toes are higher than the head and that the body is in a V-shaped position. Reach your arms forward towards the legs, keeping them as straight as possible through the fingertips.

As you lift your legs, feel your tailbone rooting towards the floor. Relax the shoulders away from the ears by spreading the shoulder blades wide, but try not to round through the back or strain forward with the neck. Tuck the chin slightly to keep the neck long and in line with the spine. The bodyweight should be evenly distributed between the tailbone and continue breathing for a few moments. You should feel the muscles of the abdomen and the deep hip flexors working in this posture.

Variations:

Modified Boat: If you have knee problems, or are unable to straighten your legs for any reason, when you lift your feet off the mat, keep your knees bent at a ninety-degree angle. Raise the knees and feet to chest level and reach the arms and fingertips forward (though if you need, you may keep your hands on the floor). Again, make sure you are not rounding through the back or straining with the neck.

Dynamic Boat: You can make this pose more dynamic by lowering the legs and the torso two inches above your mat, then raising back up into boat pose. Repeat for as many reps as you can.

Modifications: If you are having difficulty keeping the legs straight and the torso from rounding, perform variation 1, but loop a strap around your feet. Pull the torso up so that the back is flat, the shoulders are dropped and broad, and the tailbone and seat bones are rooted into the floor. If you have any type of neck or shoulder injury, you can perform this pose near a wall. The wall will support your head as you lean the torso back and lift the legs.

Benefits: This pose is wonderful for strengthening the entire core, especially the abdomen, spine, and hip flexors. This pose is also wonderful for massaging and stimulating the internal organs because of the slight compression of the torso. It really works on the kidneys, and the intestines. It also provides good stimulation for the prostate and thyroid glands.

Avoid this Pose If: You have diarrhea, asthma, cardiovascular problems, insomnia, low blood pressure, or menstruation.

2. Hover Pose

Start in the plank position. Your arms should be extended, the toes tucked, and the entire body in one line. Make sure your hands are directly underneath the shoulders, and your feet are slightly closer than hips distance. Slowly bend your elbows until they are at a ninety-degree angle and pressed in to the side of your body. Keep your toes tucked and allow the heels to press away from you, creating a nice stretch and keeping the length in the back body. The entire body should be in one straight line, including the neck (your gaze should be about 6 inches in front of you). Relax the shoulders down and away from the ears. The whole body, especially the triceps and the abdomen, are working to keep you hovering just a few inches off of your mat. Keep the core activated to ensure that you are not sagging in the center of your body.

Variations:

Chaturanga with Leg Lift: Once you are in chaturanga dandasana, you may try lifting one leg and then the other for a few seconds to give yourself an extra challenge.

Standing Variation: Standing against a wall, place your hands directly in line with the shoulders. Bend the elbows until they are at a ninety-degree angle, doing your best to keep them pressed into your sides.

Variation 3: Keeping the lower body on the floor, bend the elbows at ninety-degrees and tuck the toes.

Modifications: To modify this pose, you may release your knees to the mat but the rest of your body should stay the same. In other words, use your tricep strength to keep the chest and pelvis hovering above the mat. If you're still working on building strength, you may also widen your arms so that the elbows are now away from your body, similar to a pushup position.

Benefits: This pose works the entire body. It strengthens and sculpts the wrists, the shoulders, the triceps, the legs, and the core (the abdominal and back muscles).

Avoid this Pose If: You have any wrist, shoulder, or toe injuries, or if you are pregnant.

3. Chair Pose

Standing with your legs together, look down at your feet. Turn the toes in slightly so that the big toes and knees touch and the heels slightly turn out. From there, bend your knees and sit your hips back as if you are going to plop down on an imaginary chair. Inhale and reach the arms up over your head, keeping the biceps pressed against the ears. Relax the shoulders down the back so that the chest reaches forward, creating a slight arch in the spine. Draw the navel in and up to keep the core completely active.

Variations:

Chair Twist: Bringing the hands to prayer, revolve the torso towards the left and hook the right elbow on the outside of the left knee. Continue to spin the chest up towards the ceiling, gazing up if you can. After a few moments, release the chair twist and go to the other side, hooking the left elbow on the outside of the right knee.

Figure Four: Lifting the right foot off the floor, cross it over the left knee, creating a figure four. If you can, sink the hips down even further, creating a wonderful stretch through the glutes. Without straightening the legs all the way, release the right foot down and switch sides.

Awkward Chair: Stand with your feet less than hips distance apart. Be sure to keep your spine completely straight and in one line as you lift the heels to come up onto the balls of your feet. Lift the arms up in front of you so that they are parallel to the floor. Bend the knees as low as you can while balancing on the balls of the feet. When you're ready, straighten the legs, and lower the heels down to release the pose.

Dynamic Chair: You can make this pose dynamic by entering into the chair pose. When you exhale, sweep the arms down towards the floor and straighten the legs into a forward fold. Inhale, bend the knees and sweep the arms up, moving back into chair pose. Continue for as many reps as you can, making sure to connect the breath to the movement.

Modifications: Having joint pain may affect your ability to perform this pose. If you have knee or back pain, you may do this pose against a wall by leaning your entire back on the wall and bending the knees. If it feels comfortable for you, you may lift the arms overhead, or extend them out to the sides. If you have tight ankles, you may roll up a small towel and stand on it. This gives the floor a slight lift so that you won't have to strain the calves or ankles.

Benefits: This pose strengthens the ankles, knees, thighs, and abdominal muscles. It also strengthens and lengthens the muscles of the back, and slightly stretches the chest. This pose also helps to alleviate the symptoms of flat feet, and helps to massage the internal organs of the abdomen.

Avoid this Pose If: You are suffering from any knee injuries.

4. Upward Plank (Purvottanasana)

Begin seated on the floor with your legs extended in front of you. Leaning back slightly, place both hands on the floor directly underneath the shoulders, fingertips facing towards your toes. Simultaneously pushing through the hands and contracting your seat, lift the hips until the soles of the feet are flat on the floor. Continue pushing the floor away with your hands, lifting through the chest and the hips. Let the head drop back to get a deep stretch in the throat. Hold the pose for as long as possible before releasing the seat back to your mat.

Variations:

Modified Plank: If you have neck, wrist, or shoulder problems, you may practice the seated version of this pose. Keeping your seat and hips on the floor, lean back slightly and place your hands on the ground with your fingertips facing towards your toes.

Table Top: If you have very tight shoulders, this is a great variation. Starting from a seated position, bend your knees and bring the soles of your feet to the mat while simultaneously placing your hands behind you, fingertips facing towards the toes. Contract through the glutes and lift the hips up off the floor. You should be exerting equal pressure between the hands and the feet, pressing away from the mat to keep the torso lifted. If flexibility allows, you

Modifications: If you have any neck or shoulder injuries, you may do this pose with the support of a chair under your head or against the wall.

Benefits: This pose builds heat in the body. It is the counter-pose to chaturanga in that it opens the entire front body, especially the chest, throat, shoulders, ankles, and arms. It's also beneficial for the wrists, the gluteus muscles, and the legs.

Avoid this Pose If: You have any wrist injuries.

5. Sun Salutations (Surya Namaskara)

Sun salutations are made up of a series of poses made to prepare the practitioner for all of the poses later in class. It is usually performed at the beginning of class to help everyone warm up and open the body. Starting in mountain pose, inhale and sweep the arms up (adding a little backbend if possible). Exhaling, bend from the hips into uttanasana, or forward fold. Step the right foot back, releasing the knee to the floor. There, reach the chest forward and look up if you can. After a few breaths, Step the left foot back to meet the right in plank pose. Release the knees to the mat, then your chest, then your chin. Breathe here and feel the arch in the lower back as you surrender your heart completely to the ground. Inhaling, slide forward to cobra pose, and then exhaling, lift the hips back into a downward facing dog. From down dog, step the right foot forward between the hands, keeping the chest lifted and allowing the hips to sink down and forward. Step the left foot forward to meet the right in a forward fold. Finally, inhaling, bring the palms together and sweep the arms up into an upward salute and exhaling the hands to prayer. Repeat this sequence on the left side. For maximum benefit, you should do at least three rounds of sun salutations daily (doing the sequence on both sides one time equals one round).

Modifications: There are gentle variations of the sun salutation sequence. For one, you may start in mountain pose. Inhale and sweep the arms up and as you exhale, fold over the legs in a forward fold. Inhale, lifting the torso half way to a flat back and exhale folding back into a forward fold. Step the right leg back into a high (or low) lunge, and then step it back to meet the left, lifting the torso half way with a flat back. Exhaling, release all the way back into a forward fold. Bring the palms together and inhale as you sweep the arms up, then release the hands to prayer.

Benefits: As mentioned above, the sun salutation sequence is very beneficial for warming up the body and preparing for class. It has extreme cardiovascular benefits and stretches and moves all the main muscle groups of the body. It also increases body awareness for alignment.

Avoid this Pose If: You suffer from dizziness or are unable to stand.

Chapter 7

Poses for a Healthy Inner Body

In order to have a healthy outer body, we need to make sure our entire vessel is working properly. Yes, problems with weight may cause issues with our organs, but the way our organs function also greatly impacts how we look and feel. If the body is not working right, there is no possible way we can feel right.

All of the postures highlighted in this chapter are meant to massage and stimulate the internal organs to increase their efficacy in the body. Revolving, twisting, and bending postures provide compression that limits blood flow to any given part of the body momentarily; however, when the pose is released, a rush of fresh, oxygenated blood nourishes the organ tissue, thus enhancing its function.

Wind-Relieving Pose (Pavanamuktasana)

Lay down on your back in savasana with the eyes closed. Inhale deeply through the nose, and as you exhale, draw the navel towards the spine and bring the knees in towards the chest and give yourself a big hug, wrapping the arms around your legs and reaching for opposite elbows, if you can. You may rock side to side briefly to massage the lower spine, doing your best to keep your sacrum on the floor. Finding stillness, take a deep inhalation. As you exhale, lift the head to meet the knees. Hold the pose for 15-30 seconds before releasing the head to the mat and extending the legs out in front of you.

Variations:

Half Wind-Relieving Pose: Bring both knees in towards the chest. Continue breathing and lengthening the spine along the floor. After a few moments, hug the right knee in and extend the left leg all the way out in front of you. Lift the head to meet the knee, and hold there for a few moments. Release the head to the mat and switch legs, hugging the left knee in and letting the right leg extend out. Repeat on the other side.

Modifications: If you have very tight shoulders and are unable to hug yourself comfortably, you may grab behind the knees, around the backs of the thighs.

Benefits: This pose massages and stimulates the digestive tract (especially the ascending and descending colons). Due to this massage and stimulation, this pose helps to eliminate trapped gases, ease acid reflux, and It also stretches through the hips and helps to relieve tension in the lower back.

Avoid this Pose If: You've just had recent abdominal surgery or a hernia, or if you are suffering from diarrhea.

Seated Spinal Twist (Ardha Matsyendrasana)

Begin sitting on your mat with your legs extended out in front of you. Bring the sole of your right foot to the mat as you bend your right knee. Cross the foot over the left leg so that the right foot is on the outside of the left knee. Be sure that the foot is flat on the ground. If it is not, you may need to slide it down towards the outside of the left calf muscle. Inhale and lift your arms above your head. As you exhale, drop your arms so that the left arm hooks over the outside of the right knee and the right arm plants itself right behind you. Keep lifting through the spine as you try to keep your hips pressed evenly into the floor. Use your breath as a tool to inhale and lengthen the spine, and exhale, deepen the twist. After a few moments, switch your legs and repeat on the other side.

Variations:

Half Lord of the Fishes: Follow the instructions for ardha matsyendrasana. Once your right foot is on the outside of your left knee, you may bend the left leg in so that the left foot ends up on the outside of the right hip. Proceed with the twist as usual. Eventually, switch sides and repeat.

Modifications: If this pose is not possible for you, you may let the right knee fall out to the side so that the sole of the right foot is pressing against the left inner thigh. Inhales and lift the arms and proceed with the twist as usual.

Benefits: The rotation of this pose compresses the organs of the abdominal cavity, namely the liver and the kidneys, which increases their efficacy. This pose also improves digestion, and helps to alleviate the symptoms of sciatica, and reduces the physical pains of menstruation.

Avoid this Pose If: You have a back or spinal injury.

Cow Face Pose (Gomukhasana)

Begin in a seated position with your legs extended out in front of you. Bend the left knee into a figure four with the left foot on the outside of the right hip. Bend the right knee, and stack it directly on top of the left. The right foot should be on the outside of the left hip. Inhale deeply to elongate the spine and stay lifted through the chest. As you exhale, extend your arms out to the side, fingertips on the floor, and hinge forward from the hips until you are as low as you can go. When you lift the torso, switch the legs and repeat.
Variations:

Cow-Face Pose with Shoulder Stretch: Stack your knees one on top of the other (if available). With the spine tall and straight, bend your right elbow behind your back so that the palm is facing out.

Lift the left arm and bend the elbow behind your head so that the left palm is facing in and is reaching for the right hand. If you can, clasp your hands behind your back. Keep the spine tall and straight. If you'd like a deeper stretch, you can use the head to push the left arm back slightly and open the shoulder.

Cow-Face Pose with Shoulder Stretch and Forward Fold: For variation 2, follow all of the steps for variation 1, but hinge forward from your hips folding on top of the legs until you are as low as you can go.

Modifications: You may sit in a comfortable cross-legged position if it is not possible to stack the knees. Also, for variation 1, if you cannot clasp your hands, you may use a strap or a towel, or you may grab for your shirt.

Benefits: This pose massages and stimulates all of the internal organs in the abdominal cavity. It also helps to open and decompress the lower spine.

Cow face pose is wonderful for the joints, as well. It opens the hip joints and increases their range of motion, alleviates chronic knee pain, and stretches the shoulders, ankles, and hips. If performing variation 1 or 2, it also helps to clear and open the chest.

Avoid this Pose If: You have serious neck and/or shoulder injuries/pain, if you have untreated herniated disks and the spine, if you have severe knee problems, or if you are pregnant (just forgo the fold during the first trimester).

Thunderbolt Pose (Vajrasana)

Come to a kneeling position, sitting on your heels. Keep the tops of the feet flat on the floor and do your best to keep the thighs and knees together. Place the palms on top of the knees; take a deep inhale and as you exhale, feel yourself relax into the pose. Double check to make sure your head, neck, and pelvis are all in one line. Close your eyes and breathe.

Variations:

Hero's Pose: You may separate your heels so that they are still right alongside your buttocks and hips, and let the seat sit flat on the floor.

Modifications: If you need, you may place a rolled up blanket underneath the shins, ankles/feet, or knees for some extra cushion. You may also place a block or thickly folded blanket under your seat for extra assistance.

Benefits: This is a wonderful stretch for the lower half of the body, the quadriceps, ankles, and shins, especially. This pose also increases blood flow to the pelvis and the digestive tract, which is especially helpful for ulcers, acidic gastric conditions, and acidic gastric conditions.

Avoid this Pose If: You have chronic and severe knee pain. Also, if you've had any recent surgeries on the lower body (legs and waist), do not do this pose.

Revolving Triangle (Parivrtta Trikonasana)

Begin standing at the top of your mat with your feet together. Gently step your right foot back behind you about 3.5 feet. Turn your right foot so that it is perpendicular to your left foot (which should be facing forward). Your hips should be open and square to the right side. With a big inhale, lean back towards the right leg, creating space in the ribs. As you exhale, revolve the torso and hinge forward over the left leg. If you can, place your right hand on the floor beside your left foot. If that is not a possibility, let the hand rest wherever it lands on the leg (just not on the kneecap, either above or below it). Inhale and lift the torso. Step your feet together at the top of your mat; when you're ready, step the left foot back and repeat on the other side.

Variations:

Revolved Half Moon: Keeping the arms exactly the same, you may slowly lift your back leg off the ground.

Modifications: If you have very tight leg muscles and your back heel keeps lifting, you may do this pose with the back heel rooted against the wall to make sure it stays down, but remember if you take this variation, you may not be able to go as deep into the pose, so be aware of your body and when certain tension may become too much.

Benefits: This pose also massages the abdominal organs, such as the liver, the intestines, gallbladder, and stomach. The twisting motion helps to alleviate constipation, sciatica, and chronic lower back pain. This pose also opens the chest, stretching its muscles and making breathing easier.

Avoid this Pose If: You have low blood pressure, insomnia, diarrhea, or migraines.

CHAPTER 8

CHARACTERISTICS OF YOGA

Let's take a look at some of the chief characteristics of Yoga.

1) Yoga is not an exercise.

To understand the concept of Yoga one must keep in mind that the positions in Yoga are not exercises but bodily stretches and maintenance of stretches. You may describe Yoga in terms of Yogic stretches or Yogic practices.

Acquiring a body position by stretching the muscles and then maintaining this position as long as one's body allows, that is what Yogic stretches are.

Yoga requires very smooth and controlled motions and a slow steady tempo. To achieve this one needs to have total concentration of mind while doing Yoga. The movements in Yoga are smooth, slow and controlled.

Comparison with others is greatly discouraged. Doing something beyond one's capacity just out of competition generally results in hurting one's body and hence is greatly discouraged. Breathing in Yoga remains steady unlike many aerobic exercises.

Yoga is also Isotonic unlike bodybuilding exercises, which are isometric in nature. In isotonic stretches, length of the muscles increases while tone stays the same as opposed to the isometric exercises in which length of the muscles stays the same while the tone changes.

In Isotonic stretches, body is stretched in a particular manner and maintained that way for some time.

2) Longer maintenance and fewer repetitions (as per the body's capacity).

Benefits of Yoga are enhanced with the maintenance of a body stretch. Longer the maintenance better will be the effect. However one cannot force oneself into maintaining the stretch longer than the body can bear.

Each and every position is pleasant and stable (Sthiram Sukham Asanam). Sthiram means steady. Sukham means pleasant and Asanam means a body posture or position. The right position for you is that in which your body remains steady (sthiram) and which is pleasant and comfortable to you (sukham).

The moment a stretch becomes unbearable and uncomfortable and the body starts shaking, one needs to come out of that position in a very slow, smooth and controlled manner. There will be more repetitions and shorter maintenance for a beginner.

With more practice, the repetitions will be fewer and maintenance will be longer. After doing Yoga one should only feel pleasant and fresh and nothing else. If you feel tired or fatigued or any part of your body aches, it only means that you have tried beyond your capacity.

3) Trust your body. Apply minimum efforts:

With the practice of Yoga, you also learn to trust your body's capacity to progress in terms of flexibility without conscious efforts. As long as the aim is in mind and the body is stretched only to its current capacity, the flexibility develops on its own.

One needs to just focus on breath, focus on the present state of the body pose and enjoy that pose as long as it feels comfortable. 'Prayatnay Shaithilyam' means minimum efforts.

Although there is an ideal position described and desired for each asana, no one is forced into attaining the ideal position. Yoga is done with the trust that flexibility is acquired after a continuous and regular practice.

There is a message here and that is to have faith in the unknown. This message along with the improved endocrine function, better muscle tone, calmer mind and increased positive outlook can be enormously beneficial for recovery from any illness.

4) Focused stretching:

The ability to stretch or pressure one muscle group while relaxing the rest of the body is called focused stretching. For example if a particular Asana is based upon stretching the stomach as the main muscle group (the pivotal muscles), then the rest of the body is relaxed while the stomach is stretched or pressured.

One has to watch for unnecessary straining of those muscles that are supposed to be relaxed. Initially this is hard to follow nevertheless it becomes easier with some practice. This habit of differentiating between different muscles for the pressure becomes very useful in other areas of life too.

It enables you to relax better while driving during rush hour. While doing normal daily tasks it makes you aware of the unnecessary tension on different parts of your body. You are watchful even while talking to someone or while brushing your teeth or when stuck in a traffic jam.

You learn to ask yourself, 'Am I holding my breath, are my shoulders tense, is my neck stiff, are my fingers curled?' etc. etc. These acts are unnecessary and they dissipate energy. Yoga teaches you how to relax and gives you time free of worries and regrets, impatience and anxieties.

5) Breathing:

Monitoring your breathing is an integral part of Yoga. Common mistakes such as holding of breath or breathing deliberately occur during Yoga. Both these mistakes must be avoided. Holding back on breath gives headaches, fatigue and thus the benefits of Yoga are lost by improper or inadequate breathing.

6) Anantha Samapatti (Merging with the Infinite):

Ultimate goal of Yoga is the amalgamation of self into the greater self. Yuja means to combine or to connect. A connection of Atma and Parmatma is the merging of the body and the spirit. Yoga is a way of life. It's a total integration.

According to Patanjali (founder of Yoga), two things define Yoga postures; a stable and comfortable body posture and Anantha Samapatti. Therefore you cannot separate bodily postures from meditation.

In fact a body that has become flexible and steady through practice of various positions becomes a good basis for the ultimate transcendental state of mind (Samadhi).

The kriya (cleansing processes) purify the body. Mudra and bandha bring the necessary stability of mind and concentration, initially on one's breathing (pranadharana) and then on God (Ishwarpranidhana). Initially the mind wanders a lot and that's o.k. One should let it wander.
Later one should count his breaths and should observe the inner and outer flow of air through the air passages. (pranadharna). This will enable him to concentrate better on himself (sakshibhavana).

In the beginning it will be difficult to concentrate since the body postures are not that steady. But with practice it becomes better and better. For this one must purposely take away his mind from body posture and focus it on to the breathing process (pranadharana).

Chapter 9

Losing Weight through Yoga

Regularly practicing yoga can certainly help make you feel better about your body. It increases your strength, makes you more flexible and helps tone your muscles as well. However, many people do use it as a means of safely losing weight. Not a lot of people are aware of the fact that yoga can help you shed any excess pounds you may have put on. However, does it really work?

The thing that most beginners need to know about losing weight through yoga is the fact that there are many different varieties of it. There are lighter varieties of the practice designed to calm the body and clear the mind. Whilst these can help in some way, you need to practice them in conjunction with other forms of exercise such as jogging, walking and aerobics. Of course, a healthy diet is a must as well.

You can also find vigorous forms of yoga that can provide you with a better workout if your ultimate goal is to lose weight. These are more advanced forms of the practice and before you start doing them, it is recommended that you go through the basics first. In doing so, you can help minimize the risk of injuries.

The most athletic yoga styles fall under the vinyasa or flow category. These styles start with fast-paced poses known as "sun salutation" which is then followed by a steady flow of standing poses. This style will keep you moving. As you get warmer, backbends and deeper stretches are introduced. Some of the most popular Vinyasa styles of yoga include:

- **Ashtanga:** This particular type of yoga is very vigorous and its practitioners are often the most dedicated yogis. If you are a beginner, it is highly encouraged that you sign up for group classes as this would help motivate you to continue practicing it. The series of poses are quite easy to learn and once you are familiar with them, you can take your practice at home.

Poses:

The primary series is what is often referred to as the Yoga Chikitsa. It is intended to help in realigning the spine, build strength, detoxify the body as well as boost stamina and flexibility. This is a series comprised of about 75 poses and usually takes an hour or two to complete, depending on how familiar you are with it.

The next series is referred to as the Nadi Shodana and it helps with strengthening as well as cleansing the nervous system, along with all the other subtle energy channels in our body. The last four series, also considered as more advanced yoga varieties, are called Sthira Bhaga. This means divine stability and focuses more on difficult arm balances that require a lot of practice should beginners try and attempt to perform them.

For the most part, people do skip this particular stage in the progression but if you're keen on both improving your level as a yogi and getting the workout that you need then you can give it a try.

Is Ashtanga right for you? Whilst it is quite popular, attracting students from all levels of the practice because of its athletic and vigorous style, it certainly is not meant for everyone. Trying it should help you assess if the poses are something you can pull off. The style appeals, particularly, to those who prefer doing this independently and who appreciate a sense of order in how they work.

- **Power Yoga:** This refers to a fitness-based approach to the traditional Vinyasa style of yoga. Often referred to as "gym yoga", the practice was actually molded after the Ashtanga method but differs in that power yoga does not follow a set series of poses. This can make every class unique and keeps things interesting for the practitioner. It places emphasis on improving strength as well as flexibility, with weight loss being a common result of regular practice as well.

The style can range from gentle stretching to more intense, flowing styles. This dynamic can really give the body quite the workout and certainly provides the more athletic people with a challenge.

Is power yoga for you? The practice can vary from one teacher to the other and more often than not, it appeals to the people who are already physically fit. However, if you are keen on challenging yourself whilst losing weight, this might be the right fit. There are minimal amounts of meditation and chanting when it comes to power yoga so if you are only looking for action then this is the practice for you.

- **Hot Yoga:** This particular type of yoga refers to classes done in a heated room. The temperature is often maintained at around 95 to 100 degrees, providing practitioners with a continuous and even warmth throughout the entire session. Typically, hot yoga follows a vinyasa style of movement wherein the instructor provides students with a series of linked poses to follow. The added element of heat actually makes this one of the more vigorous yoga sessions and certainly helps when it comes to weight loss.

Is hot yoga right for you? Many people tend to ask this question, considering the fact that this particular style of yoga is quite vigorous compared to other forms. The answer depends on your preferences and abilities. Given the additional element of heat, you may want to start slow and leave hot yoga for later. This should allow you to gradually move up and prepare yourself as the poses get more advanced.

Alright, so now that we've covered the basics of the three best yoga varieties for weight loss, let's take a closer look at each and go through some of the fundamental poses to help you get started!

YOGA FOR BODY SHAPE

Downward-Facing Dog

Starting at the mountain location, reach your hands to the floor and bend your knees, if necessary. Move from three or four meters before your toes with your hands extended. Push your palms, raise your hips into the sky, and press them back into your heels to make them flat (keep a slight curve in your knees to make your heels closer to earth) Keep your eye on your beings and press your chest to the thighs to build a lovely flat back.

Benefits: Stretches out the elbows, hamstrings, thighs, knees, and arches; tones and strengthens the arms and legs.

Plank Pose

Leave your tiptoes up from the downward dog and turn them, get in a high push-up spot. Put

your braces right under your shoulders, lift your heels toward the sky, and lower the hips and conform to the rest of your body. Hold here for a few deep blows. Keep your eyes a few centimeters, straight on with your hands, neck, and back and close your belly and hug your face.
Benefits: Enhances the pitch, abdominal wall, and quadricep of your deltoids

Forearm Plank
It Strengthens your shoulder blades and spread them away from your spinal cord as you spread the collarbones away from the sternum. Seek to hold your body straight, activate the heart, and look at your hands on the board.
Benefits: Increases your deltoids tone, encompasses all your abdominal wall, strengthens arms and legs, extends your shoulders, hamstrings, calves, and arches.
Chaturanga

Start to gradually lower your torso and legs in a straight line, a few inches above and parallel with your ground from a regular or high plank position. Take your look and the elbows to your sides and look back as you pull the pubis into the navel and widen the space between the blades of your shoulder. Ensure that your legs are committed and active while maintaining this position.

Benefits: Reinforce your arms and handles; tighten your abdomen and tone.

Cobra and Upward-Facing Dog

Start by lying on your belly, or lowering your body through chaturanga towards the ground and squeezing your palms tightly in your chest. Rollback and continue to raise your torso off and up as your hips are firmly planting in the floor to avoid injury by retaining minimal folding in your shoulders. Stay in cobra, or deeper, begin to extend your arms as you raise your thighs and knees out from the floor, press the palms and the tops of your feet, and look up to the sky to see a dog's pose upside down.

Benefits: Strengthens the back, arms, and braces; extend the chest and lungs, shoulders and abdomen, stiffening the buttocks and activating the organs of the abdominal body.

Locust Pose

Start with your forehead on the bottom, your torso sides, and hands facing up to the sky. Take a deep breath and lift your head and upper torso, arms, and legs out of the floor as you exhale. Take your legs actively when you firm your knuckles and spread your toes. Hold your eyes slightly in front of you on the table. You may opt to stand with arms that stretch down to the knees, or lock your hands behind you and put your fingers in one put, while you roll back and forth your shoulder blades and push your chest out even higher.

Benefits: Strengthens the back of your arms and legs, strengthening your vertebrae, buttocks, and legs; extends your shoulders and thighs; improves posture; enlists your muscles, abdominals.

Boat Pose

sit on your chest-facing mat with your knees and feet. Hold your body near the top, keep your hands, raise your feet, and parallel your shins. Keep your hands behind or release your thighs and stretch out your arms. Seek to straighten your legs and raise your arms to the sky for a further test.

Benefits: Back, neck and abdomen are strengthened, and quadriceps and hamstrings are enhanced.

Warrior I

Step your feet 3.5 to 4 feet apart from your mountain location. Keep your forefoot straight forward while angling your back foot to the top of your mat from 45 to 60 degrees. Lay your arms to the sky as you curve across your front knee, line your ankle directly, and square your hips with the front edge of your mat as much as possible.

Benefits: Stretches out the chest, lungs, shoulders, neck, belly, grind, arm, back, thigh and ankle; strengthens the shoulders, arm, or back.

Warrior III

Draw from Warrior 2, move your back foot, so your heel rises off the ground as you raise overhead arms to turn around, and find a high lung position. Keep your arms lifted from here as you move your weight forward, start your front leg, and raise your back straight behind you. Flex your back toes to the wall, balancing your front leg, attempting to build a straight line from your fingertips to your hands, back and forth, allowing your eye to stay on the floor a couple of inches ahead of your foot to stand.

Benefits: Strengthen your knees, thighs, shoulders, and back; strengthen your belly, enhance balance and posture.

Tree Pose

Catch your ankle from here and sit on the inside of your foot, either upon the leg above your knee or down the front of your calf, inside your standing hip. Bring your hands to a heart prayer, or lift them into the sky and make your arms branches.

Note: Make sure that your foot does not rest on your kneecap as it can cause injuries.

Benefits: Start at the mountain pose and stretch your fingers around your right knee as you draw them into the thorn. Strengthen buttocks, calves, ankles, and sine; expand the groin, inner thighs, chest, and neck.

Bridge and Wheel Pose

Lift your hips off the ground and into the sky by pressing your palms into the story. Hold 4 to 8 breaths, push the feet further and raise the bone as far as you can, or roll down your shoulder blades to shape a fist. Hold your hands together. Roll the spine back down to the surface, one vertebra at a time, as you release your hands slowly. Take a full wheel for another challenge. Start in the same position. Bend your knees, put your hands behind you, place your palms on the table, so your fingertips point to the floor, and your knees point to the sky. Press your palms, and as you lift your hips into the air, come up on top of your head. Start to raise your arms slowly as you lift your head away from the ground, remembering to lift through the chest and move your feet. Aim to hold for 4 to 8 breaths, then curl your head back into the throat, bend the elbows and start gradually lowering your body down to the ground.

Benefits: Enhance the entire back, including the neck, glutes, and hamstrings. Lie on your back, arms on your hands, bend your knees, and raise your feet on the floor to bring your heels as close to the bottom as possible.

Headstand

Bring your forearms to the floor from here and snap your fingers together. Keep your fingers intertwined, open your palms, and build a basket of hands with your heads. Just place your head's crown on the floor and snuggle the back of your head. Place your feet on the floor and take a deep inhale. Stay on your feet's legs, start walking closer to your knees, making an inverted 'V.' Hold the blades and raise them to the tailbone, lengthening the front torso. From here, you can lift one leg at a time, take both feet at the same time, or just jumping slightly off the ground. Keep breathing and keeping the headboard through the forearms, the middle, and the legs. Beginners will last about 10 seconds, and each time they exercise, they slowly adding five to ten seconds.

Benefits: Improves the overall lower body color, including your legs and lower torso; strengthens your arms, legs, and spinal tone; colors your abdominal organs.

Yoga for Stress Relief: Finding Tranquility in the Midst of Chaos

In our fast-paced, modern world, stress has become a pervasive companion in many people's lives. The demands of work, family, and daily responsibilities can take a toll on our physical and mental well-being. This is where the ancient practice of yoga emerges as a beacon of solace and rejuvenation. Yoga, beyond being a physical exercise, is a holistic approach to restoring balance and inner calm. In this comprehensive exploration, we will uncover the profound ways in which yoga serves as a potent tool for stress relief, helping individuals reconnect with tranquility and inner peace.

Understanding Stress and Its Impact

Stress is an intricate interplay of physical and psychological responses to external stimuli. It's the body's reaction to perceived threats, whether real or imagined. While stress can be motivating in small doses, chronic stress can wreak havoc on the body, leading to a cascade of physical and mental health issues. These may include anxiety, depression, insomnia, heart problems, and digestive disorders.

The Essence of Yoga: Harmony and Equilibrium

Yoga is an ancient practice that transcends the confines of a mere physical exercise routine. At its core, yoga is a philosophy that aims to unite the individual with their true nature and the universe. Yoga embraces the idea of balance and equilibrium, which makes it an ideal remedy for the overwhelming force of stress. Here's how yoga achieves this harmony:

Mindfulness and Presence: Yoga encourages individuals to be fully present in the moment. By focusing on breath and body sensations during practice, yoga cultivates mindfulness. This mindfulness helps individuals break free from the perpetual cycle of stress, which often involves dwelling on past regrets or fearing an uncertain future.

Deep Breathing: Yoga incorporates conscious, deep breathing exercises known as Pranayama. This controlled breathing helps calm the nervous system, reducing stress responses. It enhances the body's relaxation response by stimulating the parasympathetic nervous system, which counteracts the "fight or flight" response.

Physical Asanas (Postures): Yoga postures, when practiced with awareness and breath, release physical tension. Stress often manifests as muscle tightness and physical discomfort. Asanas stretch and relax the body, allowing for the release of pent-up stress.

Meditation and Relaxation: Yoga frequently integrates meditation and relaxation techniques. These practices offer a profound sense of calm and balance, reducing stress, anxiety, and promoting mental clarity.

The Yoga-Stress Connection: How Yoga Eases Stress

Yoga's impact on stress relief is multifaceted, addressing both the physical and mental aspects of stress management:

Relaxation Response: The practice of yoga invokes the relaxation response in the body, activating the parasympathetic nervous system. This counters the "fight or flight" response and results in a state of relaxation, reducing stress hormones.

Cortisol Regulation: Chronic stress often leads to elevated cortisol levels, which can be detrimental to health. Yoga helps regulate cortisol levels, preventing the negative impact of prolonged stress.

Improved Sleep: Many individuals experiencing stress suffer from sleep disturbances. Yoga promotes better sleep by reducing the mental and physical tension that often leads to insomnia.

Emotional Regulation: Yoga cultivates emotional regulation and resilience. It enhances one's ability to cope with stress by promoting self-awareness and emotional balance.

Increased Self-Awareness: Stress often arises from a lack of self-awareness and self-acceptance. Yoga encourages individuals to connect with themselves, fostering a profound sense of self-awareness and self-compassion.

Enhanced Mental Clarity: Stress can cloud the mind, making it difficult to think clearly. Yoga's meditative aspects bring mental clarity, promoting better decision-making and problem-solving skills.

Types of Yoga for Stress Relief

Various styles of yoga are particularly effective for stress relief. Some of these include:

Hatha Yoga: A gentle and slow-paced style that is perfect for beginners. It focuses on basic postures, gentle stretches, and relaxation, making it a great choice for stress relief.

Restorative Yoga: This style is all about relaxation and deep rest. It involves the use of props to support the body in gentle, passive poses. It is ideal for those seeking profound relaxation and stress reduction.

Yin Yoga: Yin yoga involves holding postures for an extended period, allowing for deep stretching and relaxation. It helps release tension in the body and mind.

Vinyasa Yoga: A dynamic and flowing style that synchronizes movement with breath. The dynamic nature of Vinyasa yoga helps individuals release physical and mental tension.

Kundalini Yoga: Known for its focus on energy and spirituality, Kundalini yoga incorporates dynamic postures, breath work, and meditation. It is effective in reducing stress and increasing vitality.

Incorporating Yoga into Your Routine

To effectively use yoga for stress relief, consider the following tips:

Consistent Practice: Make yoga a regular part of your routine. Even short daily sessions can have a significant impact.

Mindful Awareness: Approach your practice with mindfulness. Be fully present in the moment, focusing on your breath and body sensations.

Breath Work: Integrate Pranayama (breathing exercises) into your practice. Deep, controlled breathing helps calm the nervous system.

Meditation: Incorporate meditation and relaxation techniques. These can be standalone practices or integrated into your yoga sessions.

Seek Guidance: If you're new to yoga, consider taking classes from a certified instructor who can guide you in developing a practice tailored to your stress relief goals.

Summary: Reclaiming Peace Through Yoga

Yoga is not merely a series of physical postures; it is a profound philosophy that offers a holistic approach to stress relief. It works on multiple levels, from the physical to the mental and spiritual, to bring about a profound sense of tranquility and equilibrium. Stress, a prevalent and often overwhelming force in modern life, can be tamed and channeled through the practice of yoga. It is a journey that involves deep self-awareness, conscious breathing, and the art of letting go. Through regular practice, individuals can find solace in the sanctuary of their mats, rediscovering peace in the midst of chaos. Yoga provides a transformative path towards stress relief, empowering individuals to embrace a life of balance and inner calm.

Chapter 10

Understanding Stress and Its Impact on Your Body

Stress, the silent intruder of modern life, affects us all in various ways. It's essential to understand what stress is and how it impacts your body and mind before we can explore how yoga can help relieve it.

The Nature of Stress

Stress is your body's natural response to a perceived threat or challenge. While stress can be beneficial in certain situations, such as helping you react quickly in a dangerous situation, it becomes problematic when it's chronic and unrelenting. The types of stress you might encounter include:

- **Acute Stress:** This is a short-term stress response, like the adrenaline rush before a presentation.

- **Chronic Stress:** Prolonged, ongoing stress, often due to work, personal issues, or financial problems.

- **Physical Stress:** Stress on your body from illness, injury, or poor lifestyle choices.

- **Emotional Stress:** The result of emotional turmoil, such as grief, relationship issues, or life changes.

How Stress Affects Your Body

Stress, when left unchecked, can wreak havoc on your body and mind. Here are some of the ways it can impact you:

1. **Muscle Tension:** Chronic stress can cause muscles to tense up, leading to pain and discomfort.

2. **Weakened Immune System:** Stress can weaken your immune system, making you more susceptible to illnesses.

3. **Cardiovascular Issues:** Stress can contribute to high blood pressure and increase the risk of heart disease.

4. **Mental Health Problems:** Chronic stress is linked to anxiety and depression.

5. **Digestive Problems:** Stress can lead to digestive issues like irritable bowel syndrome.

6. **Sleep Disturbances:** Stress often causes sleep problems, leading to fatigue.

7. **Cognitive Impairment:** Stress can affect memory, concentration, and decision-making.

The Role of Yoga in Stress Reduction

Yoga's effectiveness in stress relief lies in its ability to address both the physical and psychological aspects of stress. Here's how yoga can help you find relief:

1. **Physical Tension Release:** Yoga asanas involve stretching and relaxation techniques that release physical tension and reduce muscle tightness.

2. **Deep Breathing:** The breathing techniques in yoga, known as pranayama, promote deep and mindful breathing, which calms the nervous system and reduces stress.

3. **Mental Clarity:** Meditation and mindfulness practices in yoga provide tools to quiet the mind, reduce racing thoughts, and foster a sense of tranquility.

4. **Physical Activity:** Yoga is a form of physical exercise that releases endorphins, which are natural stress relievers.

Yoga and the Stress Response

Yoga can alter your body's stress response. When you practice yoga regularly, your body learns to manage stress more effectively. Your heart rate and blood pressure may decrease, and your ability to recover from stress can improve. Yoga can help you navigate stressful situations with a greater sense of calm and resilience.

Understanding stress and its impact on your body is the first step in harnessing the power of yoga to relieve stress. In the chapters ahead, we'll explore specific yoga postures, meditation techniques, and mindfulness practices that can help you find tranquility in the midst of life's challenges.

Remember, yoga is not just about stress relief; it's

a holistic approach to well-being that will transform your life.

www.ingramcontent.com/pod-product-compliance
Lightning Source LLC
LaVergne TN
LVHW010219070526
838199LV00062B/4666